The Meal Plan for Life: Easy and Clean Nutrition That's Sustainable

The Dietitians' Gentle Detox

Other Works by Andrea Groon, Nutrition Andrea

Available through lulu.com or NutritionAndrea.com

- Planning Nutritious Meals in 4 Easy Steps
  Tools, Ideas, and Recipes to Make Healthy
  Eating Less Stressful

- Nutrition Andrea Cooks

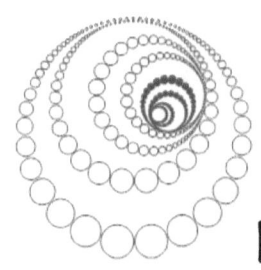

Nutrition Andrea

The Meal Plan for Life:
Easy and Clean Nutrition
That's Sustainable

The Dietitians' Gentle Detox

Andrea@NutritionAndrea.com
http://www.NutritionAndrea.com
Twitter @NutritionAndrea
Instagram Nutrition_Andrea
Facebook.com/NutritionAndrea

Contents

Introduction

Welcome and congratulations on taking the first step to a better, healthier you! Just reading this information will help you to reach your goals!

I have been helping people improve their health, increase their energy levels, and become more productive through better food and lifestyle choices for more than 25 years as a Registered Dietitian Nutritionist [RDN]. How is a RDN different from a nutritionist?

To achieve the RDN credentials, I obtained a bachelors degree (BS, Public Health Nutrition), a Masters Degree (focused on adult education and counseling) and completed a 6-month internship.

I also completed a national board exam as the final step in the process to become a RDN. Each year I must complete 15 hours of continuing education. A general nutritionist title does not include any of these educational requirements. Be sure you rely on a nutrition professional – the RDN – when making changes that can affect your health.

My clients include groups from small and large corporations as well as individuals. I also speak to large groups on a weekly basis, which allows me to reach many people at once, and it's invigorating to feel positive energy from a group of people who want to improve their health! I enjoy working directly with clients and seeing their progress, helping them through challenges they encounter, and partnering with them along their journey to achieve their goals. The results I've seen are inspiring: Often medication intake is reduced or stopped, laboratory values return to normal and overall energy levels increase. I want to do the same for you, and I hope this book will be a first step to your good health!

In this book, I will share insights on how to make sustainable lifestyle changes, using holistic methodologies and tools, as you move forward on your wellness journey. I often refer to "tools" as I work with clients. These tools are approaches, ideas, and insights that you can use along your wellness journey & for the rest of your life.

Why Are You Here?

Do you ever feel bloated, sluggish, lack energy, have dark circles under your eyes or just don't feel good? This feeling is most likely directly related to what you are eating. The old adage is true: You are what you eat. But often what is eaten has little nutritive value to our body or depletes the nutrients you do have.

If we don't put the right fuel into our body, it will not run right. Think of a car engine – if you put the wrong type of fuel into the tank, it might run okay for a while, but then it will begin to lose speed, sputter, choke out, and eventually quit running. The lines might be clogged (like our arteries or the heart), engine parts might become damaged (like the liver or kidney) and repairs will be needed (going to the doctors or having surgery). Most of us pay attention to the instructions and put the correct type of fuel into our cars to avoid these problems. So why do people put the wrong fuel into their bodies and expect them to run properly?

What The Meal Plan for Life offers you is a simple structure to make positive changes. These changes will leave you feeling energized, with healthier looking skin and ready to face what life sends your way!
Let's get started!

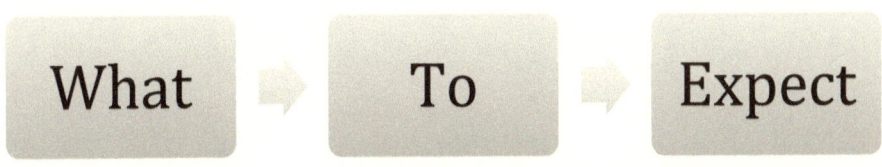

This section will outline the elements of the Meal Plan for Life and what you can expect throughout the first weeks.

The Meal Plan for Life

The Meal Plan for Life – What to Expect

You will begin by cleansing your body of artificial ingredients and sugars for four days. These 4 days will also help to reset your metabolism to fat burning levels. By detoxifying your body from these ingredients, you will eliminate food cravings. Most food cravings are driven by your body's addiction to artificial ingredients and sugar.

In the first four days, A Meal Plan for Life consists primarily of proteins, select vegetables and fats. Protein is available in many forms – both vegetarian and from animal products. Protein is complex and difficult for your body to metabolize thus increasing overall metabolism following a meal. Most forms of protein are allowed on the Plan.

Fat is needed for you to remain healthy and your body to function properly. The type of fat is the most important factor. The fats included in this Plan are natural and chosen for their specific effects. They will not lead to weight gain, when eaten according to the Plan. Most often, people eat less fat following this plan than they were previously eating. The fats on this Plan are in a different and healthier form than the fried or convenience foods previously consumed.

Carbohydrates are added back into the Plan gradually over 4 weeks, in the form of vegetables, fruits and whole grain. The order in which they are added back is designed to keep your metabolism high and body in fat burning mode.

After the first 4 days of cleansing and during the next 4 weeks, you will notice that the foods included are whole foods, which have little or no processing. The number of ingredients in any food should be limited during and after the 4-week period. Limiting the amount of artificial ingredients and sugars in your food will determine your long-term success.

You can expect to lose 4-6 pounds over the first 4 days and continue a gradual loss over the course of the plan. Most people experience a loss of up to 10 pounds after 3-4 weeks, and even more when the recommended amount of exercise is included.

You will see that The Meal Plan for Life does not ask you to count calories. It focuses on the foods your body needs to stay healthy and heal it. What does matter is removing foods that are toxic to your body and replacing the toxic foods with those that offer health benefits. Pay attention to how you feel as foods are added back into the Plan. If you begin to feel bloated, lethargic or sluggish, think about what has been added back to your diet recently. You may choose to take that food out of your plan to see if these reactions go away. Many people have food sensitivities or mild allergies that cause this type of response.

If at some point you get off track and have more than one meal of foods not on the Plan, (holiday event, vacation, etc), just start over with the 4-day detox, and then pick back up where you left off. Getting off track is not a failure or disaster – a lapse is not a relapse! Getting back to your new, healthier lifestyle is the most important thing you can do for yourself.

Activities to Maintain Throughout the Plan

Drink Fluids

In order for toxins to be excreted from the body, adequate fluid intake is another important factor of the Meal Plan for Life. The primary fluid consumed in this Plan will be water, but other fluids are also included and should be consumed throughout the day. The minimum amount to consume is 80 ounces. The suggested amount comes from this formula: take your weight in pounds and divide by 2. This number, in ounces, divided by 8 is the suggested amount, in cups.

If the number is greater than 18.5 cups – the amount suggested for a 250-pound person - use 18.5 as your goal amount. Your fluid intake should be spread evenly throughout the day – do not wait until late afternoon or any other time to drink a large quantity at once. If you include physical activity that results in sweating and lasts more than

30 minutes, add 8 ounces per 30 minutes, in addition to the base amount.

Fluids can include water, carbonated water (no sweeteners or artificial flavorings), tea (green tea preferred), coffee (no more than 2 cups per day). In later weeks on The Meal Plan for Life, wine and milk are added.

Some suggestions for reaching your fluid goals:
- Drink 16 ounces as soon as you wake up to help flush out toxins that built up overnight. Warm water with lemon juice and a dash of ginger is a natural detoxifier.
- Use a specific bottle or container that allows you to measure the amount consumed correctly.
- Use a straw to increase the amount consumed per drink.
- Use an infuser to add flavor. Oranges, lemons, limes, mint, cucumbers, etc., will all add flavor.
- Use a method to track your intake throughout the day – like rubber bands on your wrist. Put the number of bands on your wrist to match the number of 8 ounces cups you have as a goal. Each time you drink 8 ounces, take one of the bands off.
- Drink one bottle of water on your way home each day. It adds to your intake but is early enough so it should not make you get up during the night to urinate.

Stay Active

Regular physical activity is recommended to help the body clear itself of built up toxins. A combination of aerobic/cardio activity and strength training exercises will give the best result. A minimum of 2 1/2 hours per week is recommended for cardio activity. This is about 30 minutes each day, at a pace that causes you to perspire. Sweat is one of the bodies many mechanisms for getting rid of toxins. Light weight lifting or strength training should also be included at least twice a week.

The most important thing to consider when adding physical activity back into your routine is finding something you enjoy. If you do not enjoy the activity, you will not continue to participate for the long term. Continued physical activity is a large part of good health, both physical and mental. Think about what you have enjoyed in the past, as an adult or child. Some things to think about to guide your choices:

Which do you enjoy:
- Team sports/group activities or individual activities
- Structured classes or doing activities in your own time frame
- Outside or inside
- Would a exercise buddy or partner help you

There are indoor trampoline parks, skating rinks, line or other types of dancing groups, paintball groups, cycling trails, ladies only gyms (like Curves), even indoor sky diving parks that will give you a variety of options to keep you interested.

A personal trainer can develop a workout plan specifically for you or change your plan for variety. A personal trainer can be used occasionally for new, fresh ideas or used regularly if more frequent motivation is needed. Ask others for a recommendation of a realistic, encouraging trainer. If you find the trainer is not a good fit, try another trainer. Some people respond to a specific style of training (think drill instructor) while others respond better to a more gentle approach (think encouraging friend). Find what works best for you – after all you are the person writing the check! A friend or workout buddy is another great way to have support and accountability.

Yoga is a wonderful compliment to any physical activity plan and offers numerous benefits. Yoga also helps with stress reduction and managing emotions. Since stress and emotional eating is a challenge for most people, the practice of yoga gives you the benefit of lessening these feelings and decreasing the likelihood that these feelings will lead to overeating.

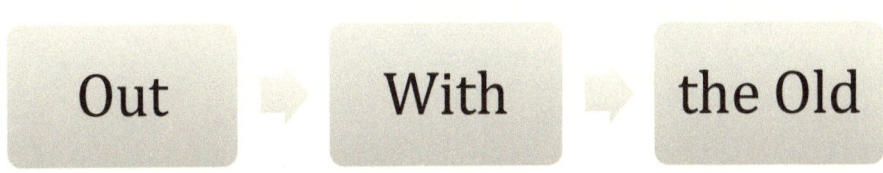

The 4 day cleansing phase will clear toxins from your body, leaving you feeling lighter, more clear headed and full of energy!

The Meal Plan for Life

4-Day Cleansing Phase – Out with the Bad (Jump Start)

The first four days are designed to cleanse your body of artificial ingredients and sugars. Your metabolism will also be reset at a greater calorie burning level that will continue day and night. Detoxifying your body also eliminates food cravings. Most food cravings are driven by your body's addiction to artificial ingredients and sugar.

In order for the Jump Start system to work correctly, you need to follow the system and eat 5 times a day (ideally 3 meals and 2 snacks). Many people are not used to eating five times a day, and most do not eat breakfast. Becoming accustomed to this frequent eating plan can be one of the most difficult parts of A Meal Plan for Life. Frequent meals are part of the design to reset your metabolism, prevent you from becoming hungry or being tempted to eat something not on the plan.

You are encouraged to be creative with the items on the Jump Start food list. Suggested menu ideas are given but as long as the foods are on the list (in appropriate amount, if indicated), try different combinations.

The Mindful Eating Tools in this book will also be useful as you begin the 4-day cleansing. Incorporating these techniques now will lead to greater success. Expect to have cravings and miss some foods – especially if you were used to consuming a high carbohydrate, sugar rich diet. The Mindful Tools, especially the ideas around decreasing emotional eating, will help you get past the cravings. Once your body is cleansed of artificial ingredients and sugars, the cravings will be completely eliminated or greatly reduced.

You may experience some side effect of the toxins leaving your body. They are normal and can include bad breath, headache, or tiredness.

Jump Start Foods
Plan to include these foods during your first four days on The Meal Plan for Life (a printable list is included in the appendix)

Protein:
Lean meat – chicken, turkey, 92% or more lean ground beef, pork roast, pork tenderloin, center cut pork chop, game meat (3-6 oz per serving)

Fish/Seafood – Canned/packaged tuna (not albacore due to mercury content) or canned wild caught salmon

Eggs

Nuts/Seeds (up to 3 ounces/day; not cashew or macadamia)
– Natural Nut Butter - peanut, almond, sunflower seed (up
to 4 Tbsp/day)
Hummus (up to 4 Tbsp/day – most flavors are okay just
check for sugar. Should be zero grams)

Vegetables:

Lettuces   Artichoke Asparagus   Avocado   Brussel
Sprouts   Broccoli   Cauliflower   Celery   Cucumbers
Edamame (up to 1/2 cup/day)   Green Beans   Kale   Leafy
Greens   Leeks   Mushrooms   Onions   Peppers (red,
green, yellow, orange)   Spinach   Squash (summer or
zucchini)   Tomatoes   Sea vegetables (wakame, kelp,
dulse flakes, arame)   Dill pickles (make sure no sugar
added)   Sun Dried tomatoes in water or oil (up to ¼ cup
per day) Roasted Peppers   Pepperoncini

Flavorings:

Lemon – juice or sliced   Lime – juice or sliced
Vinegars   Cocoa Powder(not Dutched, Dutch Processed or
Alkalized due to chemical processing)
Herbs (all but especially these detoxifying herbs): Basil
Cilantro Garlic Turmeric/Curry Rosemary   Onion
powder   Garlic powder

Fluids:

Club Soda or Sparkling Water – can be flavored if no sugar or artificial ingredients added   tea   coffee
Chia tea (unsweetened or with approved sweeteners)
Permitted Oils: up to 3 Tablespoons/day
Butter   Coconut Oil   Olive Oil   Flaxseed Oil
Expeller pressed canola oil

Healthy fats: 1-2 servings/day:
½ Avocado   10 Olives (any color)   1oz Flax seed or Chia seed   Capers

Other:
Mayonnaise (no sugar added), mustard – not honey mustard or other with sugar added

Sweeteners:
Stevia or monk fruit can be used as a sweetener. Both In The Raw and Sweet Leaf brands have no sugar alcohol added, unlike some other brands. Sugar alcohols can be very difficult for some people to tolerate. Many people experience bloating, gas, cramping or diarrhea when they consume sugar alcohols, especially in large quantities. Sugar alcohols can be identified by the way their word ends – look for the letters – ol. Examples are sorbitol, manitol, xylitol.

Jump Start Meal Plan Ideas

Breakfast -
Scrambled eggs with spinach, broccoli or any allowed vegetables; egg omelet with peppers, onion and mushrooms; egg omelet with lean meat and vegetables. Any frittata recipe as long as it is made with allowed ingredients.

If you do not like eggs, you can select any of the meal or snacks ideas listed or create one from the foods listed.

Snacks –
Nuts, seeds, nut butter with celery, cucumber, cauliflower, hummus mixed with 2 tsp ground flax seed and pepper strips, steamed edamame, boiled seasoned shrimp, dill pickles

Lunch or Dinner -
Salad with hardboiled egg, tuna or lean meat; lettuce wrap with meat and avocado; lettuce wrap with hummus, ground flax seed and vegetable strips; lean meat with vegetables roasted, steamed or sautéed with small amount of healthy oil; grilled burger in a lettuce wrap with avocado, tomato and onions; sautéed shrimp with asparagus; Miso Soup; Vegetable Soup – can add meat if desired; shrimp salad, seafood salad, chicken salad

Name Brands – Seapoint Farms dry roasted edamame; In The Raw Stevia or Monk Fruit, Sweetleaf Stevia in liquid or powder form (any flavor); NuNaturals vanilla, liquid form, alcohol free - various other flavors available (free samples available https://nunaturals.com/page/414); Now Foods Better Stevia, packets. Duke's Mayonnaise is sugar free. Walden Farms Salad Dressing is sugar and carb free

Weekly ➡ Eats

From snacks to soups, here are suggestions for filling your plate with delicious food following your 4-day cleanse

The Meal Plan for Life

Week 1 – Begin to Reintroduce Carbohydrate-containing Foods

You made it through the first 4 days and will be experiencing few, if any cravings. You will also feel better overall – clear headed, higher energy levels, fewer GI issues (bloating, GI upset, etc).

Continue to use the Mindful Eating Tools as you develop new ways of thinking about and eating foods.
Multiple foods will be added back into the plan this week.
It is important to follow the list closely and only include the foods listed, in the portions noted.

Apples are included this week, as the only fruit. Apples are a special fruit for several reasons. They are high in both soluble and insoluble fiber (which contributes to feelings of fullness, reduced cholesterol levels and controls blood sugars) , pectin (which reduces blood sugar levels, triglyceride levels and weight), and helps to increase the number of good gut bacteria (which improves immunity and aids digestive issues).

Other items added this week, in limited amounts, are dairy products, whole grain crackers and wine.
If you choose to drink wine, a wine spritzer is a good choice that reduces the amount of sugar. Combine one of the listed wines with seltzer water in a 1:1 ratio. A splash of fresh

citrus like lemon or lime enhances the flavor and adds a healthy dose of Vitamin C, too!

When eating out, ask for all sauces, condiments or dressings on the side. Most have some amount of sugar and some have a very high amount. If sugar is re-introduced at this time, your cravings will return and sabotage your progress. Ask for your foods to be steamed with no additives. Some restaurants soak their meats and vegetables before cooking, even before steaming, to "improve' the flavor. Ask your server if this is done where you are eating and select another option if so. Remember, the least amount of processing or fewer steps involved between the raw form and it being ready to eat, the less likely the food has additives or other artificial ingredients.

Week I Foods
Foods added During Week 1 (a printable list is included in the appendix)

Protein:
Tofu
Tempeh

Fruit:
Apple
Unsweetened Applesauce (1/2 cup/day)

Vegetables:
Carrots   Sugar Snap Peas   Green or English
Peas
Beans and Peas: up to 1 cup/day
Snow peas   Chick Peas Butter Beans   Lima Beans
        Black Beans

Dairy Products:
Organic milk, soy milk, almond milk; Unflavored Kefir;
Plain Yogurt – Greek or regular, sour cream
Cheese 1 ounce/day - cheddar, feta, bleu cheese,
mozzarella, parmesan, provolone, part skim ricotta, string
cheese, Baby Bell, and Laughing Cow cheeses.
Cottage cheese, ½ cup

Grains:
Crackers: 1 Serving/day
Name Brands
Original Triscuit   Finn Crisp Hi-Fibre   Brad's Raw
Flax Crackers
Mary's Gone Crackers - (original, black pepper, caraway,
herb, or onion)
Nut Thins

Wine: 6 oz per day - prefer Italian, French or Germany

Dry Reds
Pinot noir   Cabernet franc   Merlot
          Cabernet sauvignon

Dry Whites
Pinot blanc   Sauvignon blanc   Pinot grigio
Champagne, Cava or Sparking Wine (not Prosecco)
Brut Nature or Brut Zero

Week I - Meal Plan Ideas
(In addition to previous meal plan ideas)

Breakfast
Greek yogurt or cottage cheese, 2 tsp ground flax seed and
apple sauce with cinnamon; Greek yogurt or cottage cheese
with sliced apple; apple slices with nut butter sandwich;
any of the snack ideas

Snack:
Nut Butter on crackers; Laughing Cow cheese with
crackers; hummus with carrots, celery and sugar snap peas;
apple with cheese; chocolate cottage cheese chia pudding
(see recipe in Appendix)

Lunch or Dinner:
Baked salmon with roasted carrots and asparagus; Stir fried
sugar snap peas, broccoli, cauliflower and diced chicken;
baked chicken topped with provolone, diced tomatoes and

roasted Brussels sprouts; vegetable bean soup; homemade chili; homemade cream of broccoli (or other vegetable) soup

The Meal Plan for Life

Week 2 Foods – More Fruit

This week you will see the addition of more fruit, and therefore natural sugars, back to the plan. After detoxifying your body, and taste buds, from sugars, you should notice the intense sweetness of the fruits.

Other additions this week are popcorn, sweet potatoes and beets! All of these will have portion limits.

Foods added during Week 2 (a printable list is included in the appendix)

Fruits: up to 2 cups/day
Berries – blueberry, strawberry, raspberry, blackberry, grapefruit, honeydew melon, cantaloupe

Vegetables:
English peas, Sweet Potato, beets, spaghetti squash – up to ½ cup 4 times/week on different days
Beans and Peas: up to 1 cup/day
Kidney beans, pinto beans, navy beans, black eyed peas, lentils

Dairy:
Low fat cream cheese (Neufchatel) up to 3 tablespoons/day; can increase total cheese to 2 ounce/day.

Nuts and Snacks:
Cashews, Macadamia nuts, Plain Popcorn from hot air popcorn popper or stove-top cooker (3 cups/day)
Dark Chocolate – up to 1 ounce/day of 60% or greater cocoa content

Week 2 Meal Plan Ideas
(In addition to previous meal plan ideas)

Breakfast:
Smoothies, yogurt with berry and flax;

Snack:
Sliced apple with low fat cream cheese sprinkled with cinnamon

Lunch/Dinner:
Chili with Greek yogurt & cheese; baked fish, lentils, sautéed vegetable blend; baked chicken with sweet potatoes and green beans; spaghetti squash with shrimp and diced tomatoes in Italian seasoning

Week 3 Foods – Whole Grains are Back!

This week, select grains and additional fruits are included. Portion control with the new foods, as well as all included foods, is vital.

Foods added during Week 3 (a printable list is included in the appendix)

Fruits:
Cherry, pears, plums, prunes, oranges (all varieties), fresh apricots, papaya

Vegetables:
No additions this week

Beans and Peas:
All beans, peas and lentils are allowed up to 1 1/2 cup/day

Dairy:
No change to previous limits

Grains: (up to ½ cup/day)

Quinoa, wild rice, bulgur, barley, buckwheat,

Nuts and snacks:
No changes

Week 3 - Meal Plan Ideas
(In addition to previous meal plan ideas)

Vegetable Bean soup with quinoa; Baked herbed chicken, wild rice, sautéed green beans and tomatoes; grilled fish, mixed squash, black beans; Lettuce wrapped burger, Cobb Salad.

Post Week 3 Foods

Most important thing as you continue your success is limiting artificial or added ingredients and being aware of the total number of ingredients –the goal is five or fewer ingredients and words you can pronounce. Common ingredients like salt/pepper, spices, water/milk, garlic, onions are not counted in the five ingredient limit. Continue portion control of specified foods from earlier weeks.

Foods added Post Week 3

Fruits:
Pineapple, watermelon and ripe bananas or plantains limit to ½ c /day. Limit dried fruit to ¼ cup/day

Vegetables: limit these to ½ cup, 3 times/week
Corn, winter squash, acorn squash

Beans /peas:
No change to previous limits

Dairy:
No change to previous limits or additions

Grains: ½ cup/day –
Rye, whole grain couscous, 100% whole wheat pasta,
brown rice, potatoes (limited to ½ cup 2x/week)
Bread – limit to 4 slices per week
Sprouted grain bread, Ezekiel Breads, oat based bread,
whole meal rye bread with kernels, 100% whole wheat
multi-grain bread
Pasta – limit to 1 cup/week of whole grain pasta
Pizza – limit to 2 slices/week of thin crust style
Cereals – Old Fashioned or Steel cut oatmeal, Fiber One,
All Bran, Shredded Wheat
Corn tortillas - up to two 6 inch corn tortillas/day

Wine: up to 8 oz/day

Nuts and snacks:
Pretzels, whole grain up to 1 ounce/day

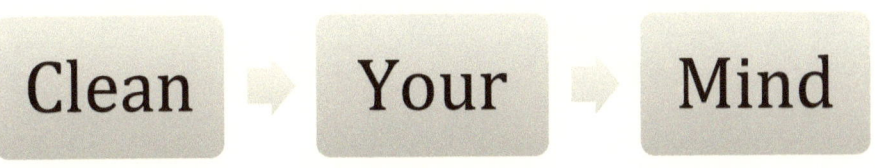

A clean mind is as important as a clean body, and will support your successful life wellness plan. These tools will empower and calm you.

The Meal Plan for Life

Clean Mind, Clean Body – Complementary Tools for Health and Wellness

Use these tools to help when struggling to maintain your healthy habits. A clean mind, free of negative thoughts and clean body, free of toxins, will help you find calm and peace, without relying on food.

The Power of Thought

Most of our thoughts are habit. Actually 40% of our thoughts are habit. When the thoughts are about us, particularly our abilities, body image or choices, the thoughts are not nice. In fact, many of the thoughts are so unkind, that we would never say those things to a friend or loved one! But we say them to ourselves and usually in a very unpleasant voice! These negative thoughts are heard so often that we begin to believe them: "I am not (fill in the blank) enough to succeed in my plan." This is called "negative bias" and unfortunately comes naturally to most people.

When we continue to have these negative thoughts, they create negative feelings, which often lead to stress or emotional eating. This acts to prove that the negative thoughts were correct: "I will not be successful in my plan because I can't resist ice cream." And the cycle continues.

Replacing negative thoughts with positive ones will break the cycle. For example: "I love ice cream and can't resist eating it." Change this thought to a more positive one: "I love ice cream and can savor a small amount as part of a healthy diet."

Go on a Media Detox

What you see impacts your motivation, confidence, and cravings more than you may know. From TV commercials tempting you with latest food creation, to magazine covers that simultaneously show size 0 models next to cupcake recipes, these messages stick in our brain. Even Facebook or Instagram feeds featuring perfectly toned professional athletes can throw us immediately into "compare and despair" mode. When our eyes and brains are assaulted with images of how we should look hundreds of times a week, it leaves us with unrealistic standards that cannot be met.

Try a 7-day media detox. Turn off the TV, talk radio programs, celebrity magazines, and anyone on social media who makes you feel bad about yourself, even for a moment. Turn it all off. By listening to your body, instead of the images forced on you, you will begin to feel better about yourself and your accomplishments. Stop comparing yourself to someone who has been surgically enhanced or retouched and airbrushed in pictures.

Toxin Releasing Cleansing Soak

This type of bath dates back many years. It helps the body eliminate toxins, relieve stress, relax tight muscles and absorb minerals and nutrients and absorb minerals and nutrients.

You only need a couple things to turn a regular bath into a detox bath. You will need 2 cups of Epsom Salts and 1 cup of Baking Soda. Soaking in Epsom salts helps replenish the body's magnesium levels. The sulfate flushes toxins and helps form proteins in brain tissue and joints. Baking soda is known for its cleansing ability and even has anti-fungal properties. It also leaves skin very soft.

You can also add other things, to make the experience more relaxing and enjoyable, like essential oils, dried herbs or even ginger.

You want the water to be comfortably hot. Soak for about 40 minutes. It takes the first 20 minutes for the toxins to leave the body and the final 20-minute for the magnesium to be absorbed. If you have any sore or tight muscles, make sure that area of the body is immersed in the water. Or soak a small towel in the water and place on shoulders or neck area.

Do not use soap or anything else until the end to allow the Epsom Salts and baking soda to function properly. Add more hot water as needed but do not drain original water or you will lose the benefits.

Take some deep breaths, sit back and enjoy! Note – if you have diabetes, consult your physician before soaking in this bath.

Avoid Abdominal Bloating

Abdominal bloating, swollen fingers and other discomforts accompany water retention. Whether you retain fluid due to hormonal changes or after eating too much salty food, don't reach for prescription diuretics. Even over-the-counter diuretics are likely to be harder on the system than retained fluid.

Instead, try the following:
- Eat sensibly and watch your salt intake.
- Get regular exercise.
- Drink black tea, eat celery or add lemon juice to your water, all safe and natural diuretics.
- Try an herbal diuretic such as corn-silk tea or freeze-dried dandelion leaf. Both are mild and nontoxic. You can get corn-silk tea in health food stores or make it yourself if you have access to fresh corn by steeping the silks in boiling water for ten minutes. Drink one cup two to four times a day. The dose for

freeze-dried dandelion is one or two capsules two to four times a day.

If bloating persists you may have a food intolerance or allergy. Consider an elimination diet focusing on elimination of one of the top food allergens at a time – gluten, corn, soy, dairy, eggs, nuts.

How to Combat Emotional Eating

5 Helpful Ways to Comfort Yourself Without Food – A Sampling of Ideas

Mindful Meditation Techniques
- Count on your senses 1, 2, 3, 4, and 5. If all of your thoughts are about food, focus on your other senses. What do you smell and hear? How does the room temperature feel? What colors you can see?, etc.
- Breathe your way to calmness. Focus on deep breaths in & out to the count of 4. Do this for at least 3 minutes.

Change Your Thoughts, Change Your Eating
- Journal about what drives you to eat for comfort.
- Laugh! Laughter engages your mind and body physically. Read a joke, look at a funny you tube video, keep funny pictures on the fridge door.
- Have a Talisman. A talisman is an object thought to have magical powers or bring good luck, traditionally beads, but can be any object that you want. You could keep seashells in your purse, pocket, or desk. When stressed, look at the natural beauty, feel the smooth surface of the shell and imagine where it had been before you found it. You can almost smell the ocean, if you close your eyes and think hard!

Calm and Relax Your Body

- Find a soothing scent. Think of a scent that brings good, calming memories and feelings. Maybe the smell of magnolia from your favorite climbing tree as a child, or your mothers perfume, or the classics lavender, eucalyptus or lemon.
- Take a bath. Hydrotherapy, like a soothing warm bath or shower, feels like it is washing away the stress and negative emotions. And gets you in a quiet space alone which will allow you to decompress.
- Get your hands busy. Find an activity you enjoy that uses your hands – knitting, scrapbooking, painting, making soap, needle point, playing an instrument or piano, etc. The goal is to keep your hands, and mind, busy.
- Challenge your brain. Play mind games like Sudoku, crossword puzzles, jigsaw puzzles, solitaire on the computer or with cards.

Social Relationships

- Find a buddy. This person is there for support, venting, and listening. They are not there to solve a problem or tell you what to do but listen and offer non-judgmental support.
- Hang out with animals. Take the dog for a short walk, play with the cat and his favorite toy or just enjoy their funny expressions and feel their unconditional love for you. If you don't have a pet,

offer to walk your neighbors or consider volunteering at a shelter.

Recipes

With just a few ingredients each and minimal prep steps, there recipes will allow you to maintain healthy eating while achieving all of your other life goals. I know you can do it!

The Meal Plan for Life

RECIPES

SNACKS

Vanilla Almond Popcorn
½ c popcorn kernels, popped
2 T coconut oil
2 dates
2 tsp vanilla extract
1 T almonds
1 T water

Combine coconut oil, dates, vanilla, almonds and water in a food processor. Pulse until smooth, scraping sides as needed.

In a large bowl combine popcorn with sauce. Toss to coat. Place mixture on a large cookie sheet and bake 8 – 10 minutes at 350°. Stir every 2 minutes, until no longer soggy.
Cool on a wire rack. Store remaining in an air-tight container.

Buffalo Ranch Popcorn
12 c popped popcorn
1 tsp granulated garlic
½ tsp dried dill

¼ tsp cumin
½ tsp sea salt
4 T butter
2 tsp hot sauce like Texas Pete
In a small bowl, combine garlic, dill, cumin & sea salt.
In another bowl, melt butter then add the hot sauce. Mix
until combined. Toss this with the popcorn to coat. Then
toss with seasoning blend.

Feta Cheese Dip
1/2 cup feta cheese
¼ c plain yogurt
¼ cup sour cream
2 tsp garlic
Pinch salt
Pinch freshly ground pepper
Blend all ingredients until smooth. Serve with vegetable
chips or use over fish and steamed vegetables

Roasted Chickpeas
2 (15 oz.) cans or 3 cups fresh chickpeas
1 T olive oil
1 tsp garlic powder
1 tsp onion powder
1/2 tsp chili powder

Preheat oven to 400°. Drain, rinse, and pat dry canned chickpeas. Toss the chickpeas with oil and spices. Spread out evenly onto baking sheet. Bake 30-45 minutes, stirring a couple of times during baking. Bake until they are crispy, crunchy and golden. Enjoy!

Roasted Pumpkin Seeds
Spread 2 cups of pumpkin seeds in a single layer on an oiled baking sheet and roast at 325° for 30 minutes to dry them out.

Toss the seeds with olive oil, salt and your choice of spices (see below). Return to the oven and bake until crisp and golden, about 20 more minutes.

Indian - Toss with garam masala; mix with currants or raisins after roasting.
Spanish -Toss with smoked paprika; mix with slivered almonds after roasting.
Italian - Toss with grated parmesan and dried oregano.

Kale Chips
Serves: 4
1 bunch of Fresh Kale, washed, stems removed and torn into bite size pieces
Olive oil
Optional: salt and apple cider vinegar

Toss the kale with the olive oil and sprinkle lightly with kosher salt [if desired]. If desired, you can add some vinegar to the oil. Place on baking sheet. Bake at 375° for 10- 15 minutes. Check and stir every 5 minutes until crisp.

Crispy Carrot Chips
Serves: 4
1 bag of fresh sliced carrots or sliced carrots [about ¼ inch thick]
Cinnamon
Nutmeg
Lemon juice

Place carrots in a bowl and squeeze lemon juice over them until damp. Sprinkle with cinnamon and nutmeg. Place on baking sheet and bake at 250° for 45 minutes.

Crispy Green Beans
Serves: 1
¼ pound fresh green beans, washed and trimmed
2 TBSP olive oil

Toss green beans with olive oil. Place on baking sheet. Sprinkle with kosher salt, if desired. Bake at 425* for 15 minutes or until crisp.

Peanut Butter Dip

Combine ¼ cup of Natural Peanut Butter with ¼ cup water in a microwave safe bowl. Microwave for 20 seconds and stir to blend. Continue to heat slowly until able to blend completely. Use with fruit slices or veggies.

Pickles and Cream Cheese
Combine equal amounts of dill pickle and softened low fat cream cheese in a food processor. Blend well, adding pickle juice as needed

Cheese Chips (limit amount intake to 10 - 3 inch pieces per day)
Cheese of your choice, 2% gives crispier chips and less fat
Parchment paper-must use parchment
Baking sheet
Paper towel

Preheat your oven to 350°. Slice the cheese into thin 1 – 1 1/2 inch squares.
Lay the parchment paper on the baking sheet and place the cheese on the parchment paper. Allow 2 inches around each square, they will spread out. Bake until bubbly and brown, about 10 minutes. Once you take them out of the oven, place the crispy cheese on paper towel and blot with another piece of paper towel. Allow to cool for maximum crispiness.

Seasoned Crackers
Low Fat woven wheat crackers (like Triscuits)
Seasoning blend (like Cavender's All Purpose Greek
Seasoning)

Sprinkle each cracker with seasoning blend. Broil on low
for 3 minutes and check. You only need to toast slightly.

Onion Soufflé
½ bag frozen chopped onion
¼ c mayonnaise
1 8 oz block reduced fat cream cheese (Neufchatel cheese),
softened
1 c Parmesan cheese
2 dashes of Texas Pete or other hot sauce (more or less to
taste)

Place softened cream cheese in a bowl, add the mayonnaise
and blend. Add the frozen onion, parmesan cheese and
blend well. Add the hot sauce, to taste. Bake at 350° for 15
– 20 minutes, until bubbling and lightly browned on top.

Zucchini Nachos
3 zucchini, sliced very thin
Olive oil spray
½ c black beans
1 tomato, chopped

1 bunch scallions, sliced thin
2 T mild onion, diced
3 oz Mexican blend cheese
Shredded lettuce
1 T low fat sour cream
2 T cilantro, chopped

Preheat oven to 450°.
Place zucchini in a bowl and spray with olive oil. Sprinkle with salt and pepper. Place in a single layer on a baking pan. Bake for 15 minutes then turn them over. Bake an additional 5-10 minutes.
Remove from pan and allow to cool on a baking rack. After 5 minutes, move to a serving platter and top with 6 ingredients. Place sour cream on top and sprinkle with cilantro before serving.

SALADS

Sunshine Salad
Serves 2
2 C slaw mix
2 C romaine lettuce, torn
½ Red bell pepper, diced
1 avocado, sliced
2 tsp toasted sesame seeds
Olive oil
Red wine vinegar
Salt/pepper

Combine slaw mix, lettuce, red bell pepper and toss. Drizzle with olive oil and vinegar and toss again. Top with avocado and sprinkle with sesame seeds.

Variety of Salad Ideas

Caesar – Romaine lettuce, kalamata olives, shaved Parmesan cheese
Asian – Spinach, edamame, carrots, red cabbage, cucumber, sliced almonds
Mexicana – Romaine lettuce, black beans, cherry tomatoes, avocado, red onion, green pepper, corn, Mexican blend cheese
Greek – Romaine lettuce, quinoa, roasted red peppers, kalamata olives, cucumber, artichoke, feta cheese

Triple R – Mixed lettuce, red onion, roasted red pepper, raisins, feta cheese, slivered almonds,

Cobb – Mixed lettuce, chopped hardboiled egg, avocado, cherry tomatoes, red onion, bacon, blue cheese

Cheesy Apple – Mixed lettuces, cucumber, diced apple, chickpeas, goat cheese

Mediterranean – Spinach, sun-dried tomatoes, kalamata olives, quinoa, red onion, toasted sesame seeds, feta cheese

Festive Fall – Spinach, diced pear, red onion, walnuts, blue cheese

Classic Spinach - Spinach, mushroom, red onion, chopped hardboiled egg, walnuts, goat cheese

Garden party – Spinach, cherry tomatoes, chopped broccoli, mushrooms, green peas, cucumbers, carrots, sunflower seeds

Anti-oxidant Blend – Mixed lettuce, diced apple, feta cheese, cherry tomatoes, chopped broccoli, walnuts

Sunny Day – Romaine lettuce, edamame, raisins, sunflower seeds, carrots, cherry tomatoes

Add-Ins in addition to all above listed items
Grilled or baked chicken, baked or roasted turkey, tofu, tempeh, chopped kale, marinated beets, cauliflower, scallions, purple onions, broccoli slaw mix, banana peppers, grape/Roma/vine tomatoes, reduced fat mozzarella cheese, Parmesan cheese, kidney beans, other beans

MAIN & SIDE DISHES

Frittatta
Serves: 6

Choose any combination of the following:
1 onion, diced
1 bell pepper, diced
1 roasted red pepper, diced
1-2 c broccoli, cauliflower, carrots, spinach, tomato, mushroom
1 c chicken, pork, or beef
1 c tofu, diced
Any other allowed vegetable

Seasoning Options:
1-3 tsp spices, like oregano, basil, thyme, smoked paprika, cumin, chili powder
1-2 cloves garlic, minced
1/2 - 1 tsp salt

Frittata Ingredients:
6 – 8 eggs
1/2 - 1 cup shredded cheese (optional)

Heat the oven to 400°F.

If the meat is raw, cook thoroughly. Remove it from the pan. Keep warm. Sauté the vegetables in olive oil over medium-high heat, starting with the longer-cooking veggies like onions and ending with softer veggies like red peppers. Layer all ingredients and warm through.

Roasted Vegetables
Serves: 4

1 pound fresh vegetable of choice, washed and trimmed or cut, if needed
Olive oil
Sale/pepper
Parmesan cheese [optional]

Toss vegetable in olive oil. Place on baking sheet. Sprinkle with salt and pepper. Roast at 375° for 10 minutes. Stir and roast for 5 – 10 minutes more. Check to make sure they do not burn. Remove from oven and sprinkle with Parmesan cheese, if desired.

Salmon & Asparagus Packets
3 – 4 oz salmon
2 T chopped onion
1 tsp garlic powder
Salt/pepper
2 T low sodium soy sauce
¼ pound asparagus, trimmed

In a foil packet, combine all ingredients. Bake at 350° for 20 minutes or until fish flakes easily.

Cilantro Sauce
Makes: ½ cup
1 jar capers
1 cup cilantro
3 T olive oil
3 T green onions, chopped

Combine 2 T capers, 1 T caper brine, cilantro, olive oil, and 1 T water in the bowl of a small food processor. Process until smooth. Serve with grilled meat, as a salad dressing, over steamed vegetables, brown rice, quinoa, or whole grain couscous.

Roasted Brussels Sprouts (or Cabbage)
1 pound fresh Brussels sprouts, washed and cut in half (or cut head of cabbage into quarters)
Olive oil
Sale/pepper
Parmesan cheese (optional)

Toss Brussels sprouts in olive oil. Place on baking sheet. Sprinkle with salt and pepper. Roast at 375° for 10 minutes. Stir and roast for 5 – 10 minutes more. Check to make sure they do not burn. Remove from oven and sprinkle with Parmesan cheese, if desired.

Squash Casserole
Serves: 6
1 lb yellow squash, diced
½ large onion, chopped
1 clove garlic, chopped
½ c mayonnaise
1 c 2% cheddar cheese, shredded, divided
1 egg
Seasoning blend

Steam squash, onion and garlic. Combine mayonnaise, ¾ cup cheese, and egg. Mix well.
In a greased baking dish, combine the squash mixture, mayonnaise mixture and seasoning blend. Top with the remaining ¼ cup of cheese. Bake at 350° for 40 minutes.

Cauliflower Pizza Crust
½ head cauliflower (about 2 cups 'riced' in food processor or purchased already 'riced')
1 red onion, diced
2 large cloves garlic, minced
1 T olive oil
1 c mozzarella cheese, shredded
3 eggs, beaten

1 T garlic herb seasoning (I use McCormick Perfect Pinch Herb and Garlic)
½ tsp oregano
½ tsp basil
1 tsp crushed red pepper flakes

Preheat oven to 400°.

Place your baking stone in the oven, or grease a cookie sheet.
Remove stems and leaves from cauliflower and chop the florets in a food processor until it is roughly the texture of rice. You can also use a cheese grater, or chop the cauliflower finely with a knife.

Sauté the 'riced' cauliflower, onion and garlic with olive oil in a frying pan over medium heat until the onion is soft (about 5 minutes).

In a bowl, mix the cauliflower mixture with the rest of the ingredients. Spread the dough evenly over the baking stone, cookie sheet or cast iron skillet. If using a cast iron skillet, make sure it is well seasoned. The crust should be about 1/4 of an inch, and no thicker than 1/2 an inch thick.

Bake for 25-30 minutes or until the crust is golden brown with crispy edges. Remove the crust from the oven and cover with your favorite toppings. Keep in mind that greasy toppings will soften or make the crust greasy, so try not to use fatty cheese or sausage.

Put the pizza back into the oven and cook for 10 minutes, or until the cheese has melted and the toppings are hot. You can also broil for the last 2 minutes to brown cheese. Allow to sit for 10 minutes for crust to firm.

SOUPS

5-minute Miso Soup
Serves: 1

Boil 1 cup of water. Add 1 TBSP miso, ¼ c sliced dulse seaweed, 2 TBSP minced scallion, I TBSP grated ginger, optional 2TBSP diced tofu. Combine and allow to blend for 5 minutes.

Cream of ANY Vegetable Soup
Serves: 6

1 TBSP olive oil
½ cup onion, chopped
4 cups chicken stock
¼ cup butter
¼ cup flour
½ sp salt
¼ tsp white pepper
3 cups skim milk

VEGETABLE CHOICES
Cream of Artichoke
2 ¼ cups artichoke hearts, rinsed

Cream of Asparagus
5 cups asparagus, cut into 2 inch pieces

1 ½ tsp lemon juice
¼ tsp tarragon leaves, crumbled

Cream of Broccoli
5 cups broccoli florets
1 tsp thyme, crushed
½ cup Gruyere cheese

Cream of Cauliflower
5 cups cauliflower florets
¾ tsp curry

Cream of Spinach
6 cups fresh spinach leaves, packed OR 3 cups frozen,
thawed and drained
¼ tsp ground nutmeg

Heat oil in a large saucepan. Sauté the onion over medium-
low heat until soft but not brown, about 5 minutes.

Add chicken stock, vegetables and appropriate seasonings.
Simmer over medium heat until vegetables are tender.
(Timing will vary depending upon the vegetable. Broccoli
and cauliflower will take longer than the others.)

When vegetables are soft, place about 1/3 of the soup
mixture in a blender or food processor and process until the
mixture is smooth. Allow the lid to vent. Repeat with the
remaining soup until all is pureed.

Stir in appropriate cheese. Cover and set aside.

Melt butter in an 8 quart stock pot over medium low heat.
Slowly blend in the flour, salt and pepper. Stir to form a
smooth paste, just until it begins to turn golden brown. Add
milk slowly, stirring constantly. Cook until mixture
thickens. Add vegetable puree and cook, stirring, until
heated thoroughly.
Serve immediately.

SMOOTHIES

Cinnamon Smoothie
½ c spinach
¼ tsp cinnamon
½ c berries, fresh or frozen
1 tsp ground flax seed or chia seed
Unsweetened milk alternative
Combine in blender and add ice to desired consistency.

Chocolate Smoothie
2 tsp cocoa powder
1 frozen banana
1 T chopped dates
1 T peanut, almond, cashew, or sunflower, etc butter
6 ounces almond milk
Combine in blender. Add ice to desired consistency.

Sweet Potato Smoothie
½ medium baked sweet potato
½ c plain 0% fat Greek yogurt
½ banana or 1/2 cup frozen berries
2 tsp unsweetened cocoa powder
3 ice cubes
Combine in blender. Add ice to desired consistency. Can add stevia or monk fruit if desired.

Morning Smoothie
½ cup mixed berries
½ banana
1 TBSP ground flax seed or chia seed
½ cup frozen chopped spinach or kale
1 cup coconut water, unflavored
1 capsule probiotic
Silken tofu, optional

Combine all ingredients in blender except the probiotic
capsule. Open the capsule and add to mixture.. Blend
adding water or ice as needed to desired consistency. Can
add stevia or monk fruit if desired. The tofu makes the
smoothie creamy.

DESSERTS

Chocolate Cottage Cheese Chia Pudding
Serves 1

1 c cottage cheese
1/3 c almond milk
1 heaping spoon cocoa powder
7 drops of stevia
2 T chia seeds

Blend first four ingredients together. The desired consistency is milky, not too thick, so if you need more almond milk, add it in tablespoon by tablespoon until you achieve a milky consistency.
Add chia seeds and stir.

Refrigerate overnight (or for a few hours if you're in a rush).

Cake Batter Chia Pudding
2-3 servings

6 tablespoons chia seeds
1 cup unsweetened almond or soy milk (plus more for blending)
6 dates, pitted + well-chopped
1/4 cup almond butter
1/4 cup rolled oats

1 1/2 tablespoons cacao nibs
1 teaspoon pure vanilla extract
1/4 teaspoon almond extract

Stir chia seeds with the milk in a bowl and add the dates, almond butter, and oats. Cover and place in the fridge for at least 3 hours or overnight).

Scoop the mixture in your blender with the cacao nibs, 1/2 teaspoon vanilla, and 1/4 teaspoon almond extract. Add a splash of milk and blend until fully smooth and creamy. Add more milk as needed (slowly) to keep the pudding as thick as possible.

Taste and add 1/2 teaspoon more vanilla extract if desired and few more small drops of almond extract. For more sweetness blend in more chopped dates (soaked for easier blending). Refrigerate in a sealed container until chilled. Mixture will thicken a bit more as it sits.

Cinnamon Nut Butter
Combine roasted nuts and with cinnamon. Process in a food processor to make cinnamon nut butter. You can purchase roasted nuts or roast your own. To roast your own, place nuts on a cookie sheet and roast for about 10 minutes at 300°, until brown & toasted.

Pecan Date Bon Bons

Makes 8 -10

¾ c pecans

½ c pitted dates, chopped

2 tsp orange zest

Pinch sea salt

¼ tsp cinnamon

½ tsp white rice miso (up to 1 tsp per taste)

¼ c shredded unsweetened coconut

Preheat oven to 300°. Place pecans on a cookie sheet and roast for about 10 minutes, until brown & toasted. Let cool.

Put all ingredients except coconut in food processor. Pulse until you have an even texture. With moist hands, roll the mixture into 1-inch balls. Spread the coconut on a place and roll each ball in the coconut, covering each one evenly.

Foods Included During Each Phase

The list of foods for each phase follows. I wanted to have it in an easily printable format so it can be posted in your kitchen or wherever you might need it to support your success.

NOTE:
When evaluating whether a food is an appropriate choice, follow these guidelines.
Allowable carbohydrate amount per serving
Vegetables – 6 grams per half cup, no added sugar
Fruit – 12 grams per half cup, no added sugar
Crackers – 20 grams per serving, no added sugar

Foods Included During Jump Start

Protein:
Lean meat (3-6 oz per serving)   Seafood
Canned/packaged tuna (not albacore) or salmon
Eggs   Nuts/Seeds (up to 3 ounces/day; not cashew or
macadamia)   Natural Nut Butter - peanut, almond,
sunflower seed (up to 4 Tbsp/day)   Hummus (up to 4
Tbsp/day)

Vegetables:
Lettuce   Artichoke Asparagus   Avocado   Brussels
Sprouts   Broccoli   Cauliflower   Celery   Cucumbers
Edamame (up to 1/2 cup/day)   Green Beans   Kale Leeks
Mushrooms   Onions   Peppers (red, green, yellow,
orange)   Spinach   Squash (summer or zucchini)
Tomatoes   Sea vegetables (wakame, kelp, dulse flakes,
arame)   Dill pickles (make sure no sugar added)   sun
dried tomatoes in water or oil (up to ¼ cup per day) roasted
peppers pepperoncini

Flavorings:
Lemon – juice or sliced   Lime – juice or sliced
Vinegars   Cocoa Powder(not Dutched, Dutch Processed or
Alkalized due to chemical processing)

Herbs (all but especially these detoxifying herbs):
Basil   Cilantro Garlic   Turmeric/Curry   Rosemary
Ginger

Fluids:
Club Soda or Sparkling Water (can be flavored if no sugar
or artificial ingredients added)   tea   coffee
Chia tea (unsweetened or with approved sweeteners)

Permitted Oils: up to 3 Tablespoons/day
Butter   Coconut Oil   Olive Oil   Flaxseed Oil
Expeller pressed canola oil

Healthy fats: 1-2 servings/day:
½ Avocado   10 Olives   1oz Flax seed or Chia seed

Sweeteners:
Stevia or monk fruit

Foods ADDED During Week 1

Protein:
Tofu, tempeh

Fruit:
Apple   Unsweetened Applesauce (1/2 cup/day)

Vegetables:
Carrots

Beans and Peas:
Sugar Snap Peas, Snow peas, English peas, Butter beans,
Lima beans, chick peas/hummus

Dairy Products:
Organic milk (skim, 1% or 2%) , ½ & ½ cream (up to ¼
cup/day), soy milk, almond milk; any unsweetened 'milk'
alternative; Unflavored Kefir; Unsweetened yogurt from
dairy or alternative 'milk' – Greek or regular

Cheese 1 ounce/day - cheddar, feta, mozzarella, parmesan,
provolone, part skim ricotta, string cheese, Baby Bell, and
Laughing Cow cheeses.

Cottage cheese, ½ cup

Grains:

The Meal Plan for Life

Crackers: 1 Serving/day of these brands - Triscuit   Finn Crisp Hi-Fibre   Brad's Raw Flax Crackers
Mary's Gone Crackers - (original, black pepper, caraway, herb, or onion)   Nut Thins

Wine: 6 oz per day - prefer Italian, French or Germany
Dry Reds
Pinot noir   Cabernet franc   Merlot
        Cabernet sauvignon

Dry Whites
Pinot blanc   Sauvignon blanc   Pinot Grigio

Champagne, Cava or Sparking Wine (not Prosecco due to sugar content)
Brut Nature or Brut Zero

Foods ADDED during Week 2

Fruits: up to 2 cups/day
Berries – blueberry, strawberry, raspberry, blackberry, grapefruit, honeydew melon, cantaloupe

Vegetables:
Sweet Potato, beets, spaghetti squash – up to ½ cup 4 times/week on different days

Beans and Peas: up to 1 cup/day
Kidney beans, pinto beans, navy beans, black eyed peas, lentils

Dairy:
Low fat cream cheese (Neufchatel) up to 3 tablespoons/day; can increase total cheese to 2 ounce/day.

Nuts and Snacks:
Cashews, Macadamia nuts, Plain Popcorn from hot air popcorn popper or stove top cooker (3 cups/day)
Dark Chocolate – up to 1 ounce/day of 60% or greater cocoa content

Foods ADDED during Week 3

Fruits:
Cherry, pears, plums, prunes, oranges (all varieties), fresh apricots, papaya

Vegetables:
No additions this week

Beans and Peas:
All beans, peas and lentils are allowed up to 1 1/2 cup/day

Dairy:
No change to previous limits

Grains: (up to ½ cup/day)
Quinoa, wild rice, bulgur, barley, buckwheat,

Nuts and snacks:
No changes

Foods ADDED POST Week 3

Fruits:
Pineapple, watermelon and ripe bananas or plantains limit to ½ c /day. Limit dried fruit to ¼ cup/day

Vegetables: limit to ½ cup 3 times/week
Corn, winter squash, acorn squash
Beans and peas:
No change to previous limits

Dairy:
No change to previous limits or additions

Grains - ½ cup/day – rye, whole grain couscous, 100% whole wheat pasta, potatoes (limited to ½ cup 2x/week)

Bread – limit to 4 slices per week
Sprouted grain bread, Ezekiel Breads, oat based bread, whole meal rye bread with kernels, 100% whole wheat multi-grain bread

Pasta – limit to 1 cup/week of whole grain pasta

Pizza – limit to 2 slices/week of thin crust style

Cereals – Old Fashioned or Steel cut oatmeal, Fiber One, All Bran

Corn tortillas - up to two 6 inch corn tortillas/day

The Meal Plan for Life

Wine: up to 8 oz/day

Nuts and snacks:
Pretzels, whole grain up to 1 ounce/day

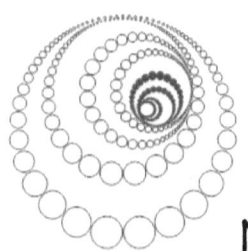

Nutrition Andrea

Andrea Groon MEd RDN, LDN
211 East Six Forks Road, Suite 202 B
Raleigh, NC 27609

Andrea@NutritionAndrea.com
http://www.NutritionAndrea.com
Twitter @NutritionAndrea
Facebook /NutritionAndrea
Instagram Nutrition_Andrea

www.ingramcontent.com/pod-product-compliance
Lightning Source LLC
Chambersburg PA
CBHW020336290526
45785CB00005B/2046

* 9 7 8 1 3 6 5 4 7 9 5 9 5 *